'Mudras for Women'

25 Simple Hand Gestures every Woman should know for attaining a Healthy Body, Beautiful Skin, Supercharged Sex Drive and Enhanced Vitality

by

Advait

TheCalmHealer.com

Disclaimer and FTC Notice

Mudras for Women: 25 Simple Hand Gestures every Woman should know for attaining a Healthy Body, Beautiful Skin, Supercharged Sex Drive and Enhanced Vitality
Copyright © 2016, Advait. All rights reserved.

ISBN-13: 978-1533342102

ISBN-10: 1533342105

medical problems without the advice of a physician, either directly or indirectly.

The intent of the author is only to offer information of a general nature to help you in your quest for emotional, spiritual and physical well being. In the event you use any of the information in this book for yourself, which is your constitutional right, the author and the publisher assume no responsibility for your actions.

Under no circumstances will any legal responsibility or blame be held against the publisher for any reparation, damages, or monetary loss due to the information herein, either directly or indirectly. The information herein is offered for informational purposes solely, and is universal as so. The presentation of the information is without contract or any type of guarantee assurance.

Adherence to all applicable laws and regulations, including international, federal, state, and local governing professional licensing, business practices, advertising, and all other aspects of doing business in the US, Canada, or any other jurisdiction is the sole responsibility of the purchaser or reader.

Neither the author nor the publisher assumes any responsibility or liability whatsoever on the behalf of the purchaser or reader of these materials.

Advait

Any perceived slight of any individual or organization is purely unintentional.

Mudras for Women

Contents

Advait

Introduction

The ancient Vedic culture teaches us that the Universal Cosmic Energy (World Energy) is made up of two halves, **Shiva** and **Shakti**.

Shiva is the Masculine component and *Shakti*, the Feminine, and women are considered as the physical human manifestation of Shakti, the one who protects, preserves and helps the world thrive.

Though the responsibilities and burdens of the world fall equally on the shoulders of women and men in these modern times, Yet by natural design, women are subjected to much greater responsibilities.

A woman undergoes three important stages in her lifetime,

Menstruation
Pregnancy
Menopause

Each of which affect her physically as well as psychologically.

That is where Mudra healing comes in, by performing these simple hand gestures, every

Advait

woman can find a natural balance between her body, mind and soul.

In this book I have mentioned the benefits of every Mudra individually, for your easy reference, along with the instructions about performing the Mudras, the duration for which they are to be performed and with well illustrated images.

If you have read my other books, you would know that I always keep my works concise and absolutely fluff-free, so that is enough introduction, let's dive in...

What are Mudras?

According to the Vedic culture of ancient India, our entire world is made of 'the five elements' called as *The Panch-Maha-Bhuta's*. The five elements being **Earth**, **Water**, **Fire**, **Wind** and **Space/Vacuum**. They are also called the earth element, water element, fire element, wind element and space element.

These five elements constitute the human body – the nutrients from the soil (earth) are absorbed by the plants which we consume (thus we survive on the earth element), the blood flowing through own veins represents the water element, the body heat represents the fire element, the oxygen we inhale and the carbon dioxide we exhale represents the wind element and the sinuses we have in our nose and skull represent the space element.

As long as these five elements in our body are balanced and maintain appropriate levels we remain healthy. An imbalance of these elements in the human body leads to a deteriorated health and diseases.

Now understand this, the command and control center of all these five elements lies in our fingers. So literally, our health lies at our fingertips.

Advait

The Mudra healing method that I am going to teach you depends on our fingers.

To understand this, we should first know the finger-element relationship:

Thumb – Fire element.

Index finger – Wind element.

Middle finger – Space/Vacuum element.

Third finger – Earth element.

Small finger – Water element.

This image will give you a better understanding of the concept:

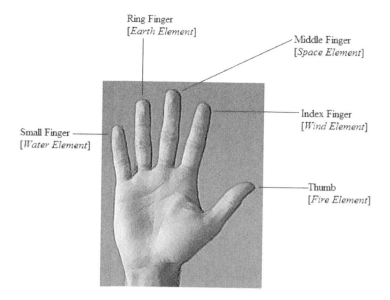

Ring Finger
[*Earth Element*]

Middle Finger
[*Space Element*]

Index Finger
[*Wind Element*]

Small Finger
[*Water Element*]

Thumb
[*Fire Element*]

When the fingers are brought together in a specific pattern and are touched to each other, or slightly pressed against each other, the formation is called as a *'Mudra'*.

When the five fingers are touched and pressed in a peculiar way to form a Mudra, it affects the levels of the five elements in our body, thus balancing those elements and inducing good health.

P.S. The Mudra Healing Methods aren't just theory or wordplay; these are healing methods

Advait

from the ancient Indian Vedic culture, proven and tested over ages.

Mudras for Women

Important

Read this before you read any further

For the better understanding of the reader, detail images have been provided for every mudra along with the method to perform it.

Most of the Mudras given in this book are to be performed using both your hands, but the Mudras whose images show only one hand performing the Mudra, are to be performed simultaneously on both your hands for the Mudras to have the maximum effect.

Advait

Mudra #1

AnaahatChakramudra / Mudra of Un-struck Hymn

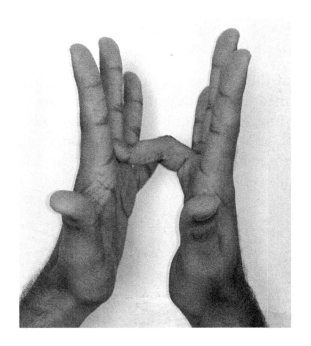

Mudras for Women

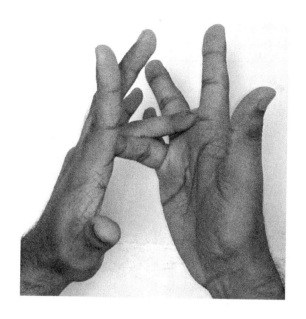

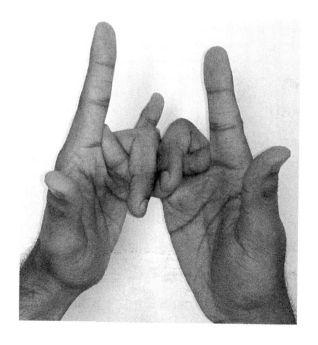

Advait

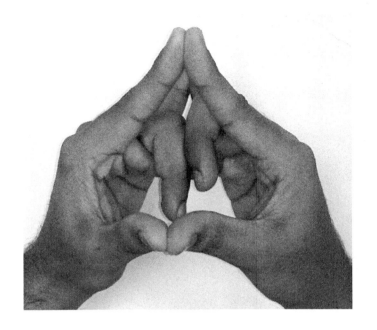

Method:

This Mudra has to be performed in a seated position.

Be seated comfortably in an upright posture and concentrate on your breathing to relax.

Place the right Ring finger on the web between the Index and Middle finger of the left hand.

Place the left Ring finger on the web between the Index and Middle finger of the right hand.

Mudras for Women

Curl down both the middle fingers to wrap and press down the respective Ring fingers of the opposite hands.

Now join the tips of both the Index and Little fingers together, outstretch them and press slightly.

Then join the tips of both the Thumbs together, outstretch them and press slightly.

This Mudra is to be held in front of your chest.

Duration:

This Mudra should be performed for at least 5 minutes and can be performed for 40 minutes at a stretch.

This Mudra should be performed twice a day, once in the morning and once in the evening for best results.

Benefits:

This Mudra enhances your body's self-healing capability.

It is an extremely useful Mudra for maintaining the health of your breasts.

It is also helpful in strengthening your Lungs.

Advait

This Mudra is known to inculcate a feeling of deep compassion and love in the practitioner.

Mudra #2

Kaaranmudra / Mudra of Cause

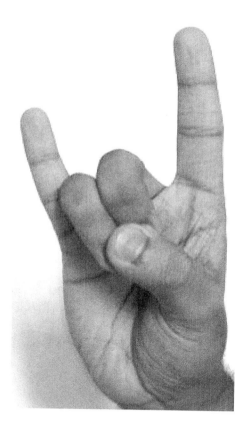

Method:

Advait

This Mudra is to be performed in a seated position.

Be seated comfortably in an upright posture and concentrate on your breathing to relax.

Cover the tips of the Middle and Ring fingers with the pad of your Thumb and press slightly.

Keep your Index finger, Ring finger and Thumb extended outwards.

Form this Mudra with each of your hand and place them in your lap.

Duration:

This Mudra should be performed for at least 5 minutes and can be performed for 25 minutes at a stretch.

This Mudra should be performed twice a day, once in the morning and once in the evening for best results.

Benefits:

This Mudra enhances the health of the pelvic organs and keeps them well toned, thus enhancing your overall sexual capabilities.

This Mudra connects your sexual energy to your spiritual energy.

This is one of the best detoxification Mudra there is.

Mudra #3

Apaanmudra / Mudra of Downward Force

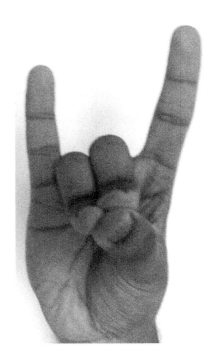

Method:

This Mudra is to be performed in a seated position.

Mudras for Women

Be seated comfortably in an upright posture and concentrate on your breathing to relax.

Touch the tip of your thumb with the tip of your middle finger and the tip of the ring finger, and press slightly.

Keep the index finger and the Little finger straight as shown in the image.

This Mudra should be performed on both the hands. Rest the hands on your thighs.

See to it that you are completely relaxed while performing this Mudra.

Duration:

This Mudra should be performed for at least 5 minutes and can be performed for 20 minutes at a stretch.

This Mudra should be performed twice a day, once in the morning and once in the evening for best results.

Benefits:

This Mudra enhances the health of the pelvic organs, thus enhancing your overall sexual capabilities.

Advait

It nourishes the Urinary bladder in both men and women.

This Mudra is extremely effective in maintaining the health of Uterus in women.

It also helps in regulating menstruation in women.

****Very Important

DO NOT PERFORM THIS MUDRA DURING PREGNANCY.

Mudra #4

AbhayHridaymudra / Mudra of Assured Heart

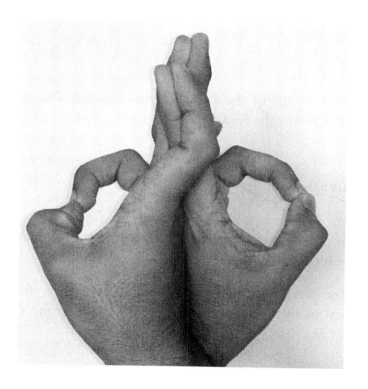

Method:

This Mudra is to be performed in a seated position.

Advait

Be seated comfortably in an upright posture and concentrate on your breathing to relax.

Join your palms together as in the Indian form of salutation 'Namaste'.

Now cross the palms at your wrist, with the back of the palms facing each other and the wrist of the right hand closer to the body.

Interlock the Index, Middle and Little fingers at the tips. (Refer the image)

Join the tips of the Ring fingers and the Thumbs as shown in the image.

Duration:

This Mudra should be performed for at least 5 minutes and can be performed for 45 minutes at a stretch.

This Mudra should be performed twice a day, once in the morning and once in the evening for best results.

Benefits:

This Mudra is very helpful in increasing your vitality.

This Mudra instantly imparts a feeling of Calmness to the practitioner. (A very useful Mudra to use when you are stressed or have just experienced a nightmare)

Practicing this Mudra also gives you more vigor if you are feeling physically exhausted.

This Mudra is also very helpful in strengthening your heart.

Mudra #5
Gadamudra / Mudra of Spear

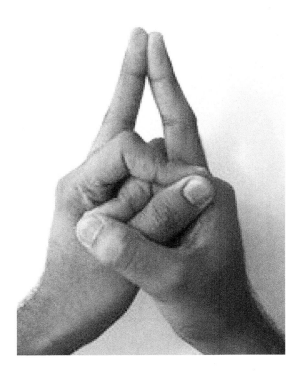

Mudras for Women

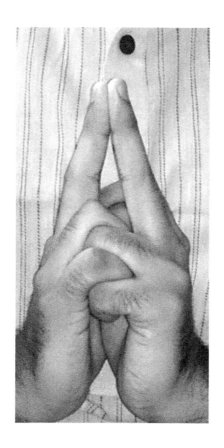

Method:

This Mudra has to be performed in a seated position.

Be seated comfortably in an upright posture and concentrate on your breathing to relax.

Form two interlacing rings by touching the tips of your index fingers with the tips of your thumbs as shown in the image.

Advait

Keep the Middle fingers straight and pointing upwards, and then touch the upright middle fingers to each other.

The final step is to interlace the ring fingers and the little fingers together, and bend them in the second knuckle such that there tips point downwards.

This Mudra should be held in front of your lower abdomen and not at chest height.

Duration:

This Mudra should be performed for at least 5 minutes and can be performed for 30 minutes at a stretch.

This Mudra should be performed twice a day, once in the morning and once in the evening for best results.

Benefits:

This Mudra is very helpful in treating hemorrhoids.

This Mudra should be performed for nourishing your pelvic organs.

This Mudra provides the practitioner with a feeling of safety and they feel protected.

A regular practice of this Mudra makes you feel well grounded and connected to the Earth.

Mudra #6

Mahashirshamudra / Mudra of The Great Head

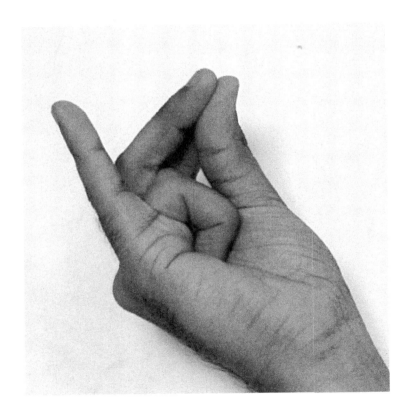

Method:

Mudras for Women

This Mudra has to be performed in a seated position.

Be seated comfortably in an upright posture and concentrate on your breathing to relax.

Touch the centre of the palm with the tip of the Ring finger.

Join the tips of the Index finger, Middle finger and Thumb together.

Keep the Little finger extended outwards.

(Refer the image)

Perform this Mudra on each hand and place the hands in your lap.

Duration:

This Mudra should be performed for at least 5 minutes and can be performed for 20 minutes at a stretch.

This Mudra should be performed twice a day, once in the morning and once in the evening for best results.

Benefits:

Advait

This Mudra is very effective in maintaining the health of your eyes.

It reduces the dark circles under the eyes.

It is very effective in treating headache.

This Mudra is also useful in relieving congestion in your sinuses.

You can use this Mudra for attaining mental clarity and calmness after a busy, chaotic day.

Mudra #7

Kapitthmudra / Mudra of Apple

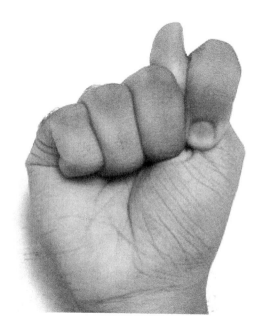

Method:

This Mudra has to be performed in a seated position.

Be seated comfortably in an upright posture and concentrate on your breathing to relax.

Advait

Insert your Thumb in the space between your Index finger and Middle finger.

Then fold all the other fingers as if you are making a fist.

This Mudra is to be made on both the hands.

The Mudra made by your left hand should be placed on your chest and the Mudra made by your right hand should be placed on your pubic bone.

Close your eyes and visualize a ray of energy entering into your chest through your left fist and one ray entering your pubic area through your right fist.

Duration:

This Mudra should be performed for at least 5 minutes and can be performed for 40 minutes at a stretch.

This Mudra should be performed twice a day, once in the morning and once in the evening for best results.

Benefits:

When regularly practiced this Mudra increases sensitivity and receptivity in the sexual organs, thus taking the sexual experience to a whole new level.

This Mudra also induces a healthy libido.

On a psychological level this Mudra can be used for healing yourself of sexual guilt and shame.

On an emotional level this Mudra induces a feeling of love, compassion and kindness in the practitioner.

Mudra #8

Prithvimudra / Mudra of Earth

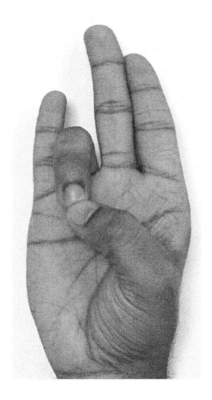

Method:

Touch the tip of your thumb with the tip of your ring finger and press slightly.

Mudras for Women

Keep all the other fingers straight as shown in the image.

(here we bring the fire element and the earth element together.)

Duration:

15 to 35 minutes, and it can be done at any time you wish.

Benefits:

Performing this Mudra regularly reduces physical weakness.

This Mudra is helpful in improving digestion.

After doing this Mudra you will feel and look extremely fresh.

If you are feeling down, this Mudra will elevate your mood.

With regular practice of this Mudra you will notice a peculiar glow of your skin.

Advait

Mudra #9

Kilakmudra / Mudra of Bondage

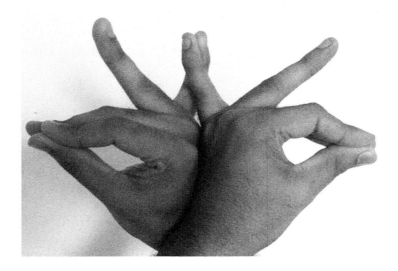

Method:

This Mudra has to be performed in a seated position.

Be seated comfortably in an upright posture and concentrate on your breathing to relax.

Cross your wrists with the back of your palms facing each other.

Mudras for Women

Now stretch out both the Little fingers, and then hook them with their tips touching and pressing against each other. (Refer the image)

Lift up both the ring fingers, slightly.

Join the tips of the Thumb, Index and Middle fingers on both the hands together.

Duration:

This Mudra should be performed for at least 5 minutes and can be performed for 35 minutes at a stretch.

This Mudra should be performed twice a day, once in the morning and once in the evening for best results.

Benefits:

A regular practice of this Mudra improves the health of your sexual glands.

This Mudra is a representative of the union of Shiva and Shakti (union of the Masculine and Feminine) hence, performing this Mudra bestows a sense of comfort regarding your sexuality and intimate relations.

This Mudra is also very helpful in improving the health of your kidneys and urinary bladder.

Advait

Mudra #10

Varunmudra / Mudra of Rain God

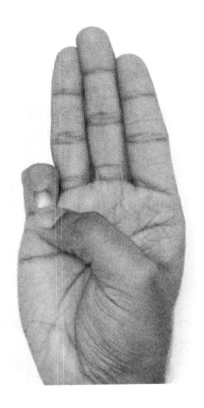

Method:

Touch the tip of your thumb with the tip of your small finger (pinkie finger) and press slightly.

Mudras for Women

Keep all the other fingers straight as shown in the image.

(here we bring the fire element and the water element together, which means we are burning away all the contamination and internal debris induced by the water element.)

Duration:

15 to 35 minutes and only when you suffer from the ailments which this Mudra cures.

Benefits:

Since this Mudra balances the water element in our body, it's a very helpful Mudra in any type of Skin disease.

Also this Mudra reduces swelling of the intestine.

If you feel any kind of itching on the skin, this Mudra will cure it.

This Mudra helps in relieving strained Muscles.

This Mudra is also called as 'Preserver of Youth'.

Advait

Mudra #11

Praanamudra / Mudra of Life

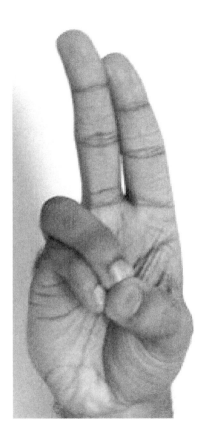

Method:

Mudras for Women

This Mudra is to be performed in a sitting position.

Be seated comfortably in an upright posture and concentrate on your breathing to relax.

Place your hands on your thighs with your palms facing upwards.

Touch the tip of your Thumb with the tip of your Ring finger and the tip of your Little finger.

Keep the index finger and the Middle finger straight as shown in the image.

Duration:

This Mudra should be performed for at least 5 minutes and can be performed for 40 minutes at a stretch.

This Mudra should be performed twice a day, once in the morning and once in the evening for best results.

Benefits:

This Mudra when performed regularly increases your physical and mental capability.

It keeps a positive stream of energy flowing through you throughout the day.

Advait

This Mudra helps regulate and ease blood flow in the body.

It is very helpful in strengthening the eyes.

It instantly relieves strained muscles.

Whenever you feel tired, practice this Mudra for 10-15 minutes, you will feel a surge of energy flowing through you.

Mudra #12

Shaktimudra / Mudra of Divine Feminine

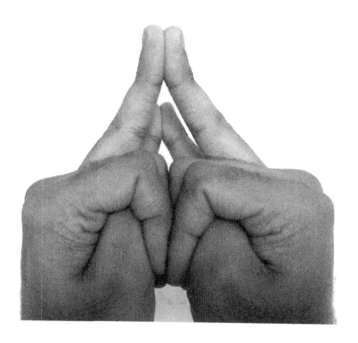

Method:

This Mudra has to be performed in a seated position.

Advait

Be seated comfortably in an upright posture and concentrate on your breathing to relax.

Keep your palms facing each other in front of your chest.

Then touch the tips of both your Little fingers and press slightly.

After that, touch the tips of both your Ring fingers and press slightly.

Fold your thumbs in to your palms

And, cover up the folded thumbs curling down your Index and Middle fingers into your palms.

Duration:

This Mudra should be performed for at least 5 minutes and can be performed for 25 minutes at a stretch.

This Mudra should be performed twice a day, once in the morning and once in the evening for best results.

Benefits:

This Mudra is works like a charm in relieving menstrual cramps.

This Mudra relaxes the organs situated in the lower abdominal region and helps you release pelvic tension.

This Mudra is also useful in treating emotional trauma resulting from sexual abuse.

A regular practice of this Mudra is known to subtly connect the practitioner with the divine feminine (Shakti) hence the name.

Advait

Mudra #13

Akashmudra / Mudra of Sky

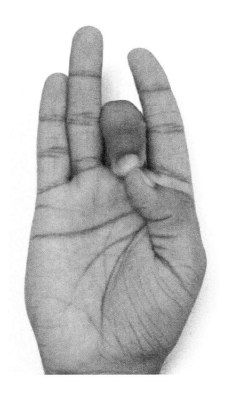

Method:

Touch the tip of your thumb with the tip of your middle finger.

Keep all the other fingers straight as shown in the image.

(here we bring the fire element and the space element together.)

Duration:

No time limit for this Mudra and it can be done at any time you wish.

Benefits:

This Mudra is especially useful for people with Heart Disorders.

This Mudra strengthens your Heart.

Performing this Mudra regularly strengthens your bones.

On an emotional level, this Mudra works as an amazing self-confidence booster.

This Mudra should be regularly performed by people with Heart disorders and Bone disorders.

Advait

Mudra #14

Yumpaashmudra / Mudra of the Death-Leash

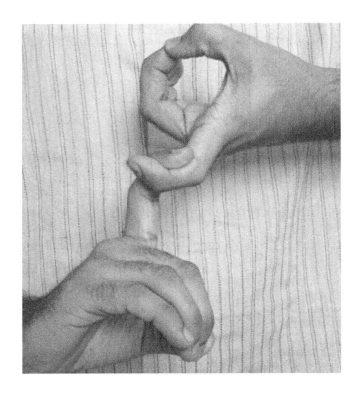

Method:

This Mudra is to be performed in a seated position.

Mudras for Women

Be seated comfortably in an upright posture and concentrate on your breathing to relax.

Extend the Index fingers on both the hands while folding the other fingers into the palms forming partial fists.

Now, hook the index fingers together, with the left hand facing up while the right hand facing down.

Hold this Mudra in front of your heart.

Duration:

This Mudra should be performed for at least 5 minutes and can be performed for 20 minutes at a stretch.

This Mudra should be performed twice a day, once in the morning and once in the evening for best results.

Benefits:

This Mudra is extremely useful in opening our nasal airways and is strengthens our lungs at the same time.

A regular practice of this Mudra enhances the immune system of the practitioner manifolds.

Advait

This Mudra is also known to induce a sense of spiritual calmness in the practitioner.

Mudra #15

MuladhaarChakramudra / Mudra of Root Chakra

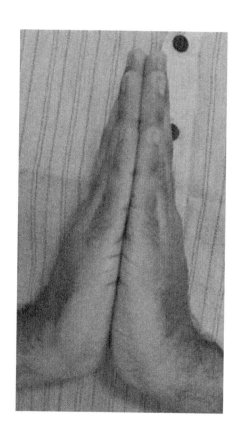

Advait

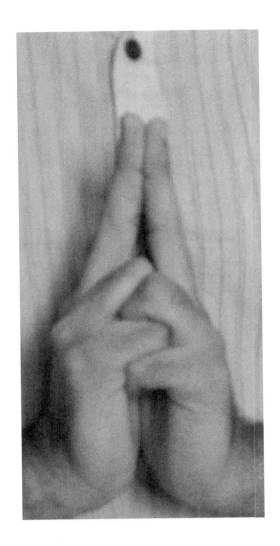

Mudras for Women

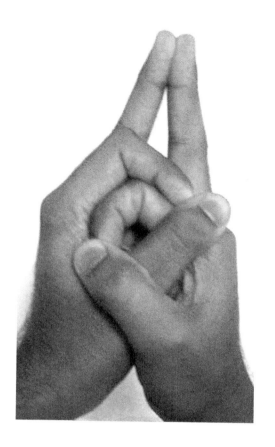

Method:

This Mudra has to be performed in a seated position.

Be seated comfortably in an upright posture and concentrate on your breathing to relax.

Join both the palms together like in the Indian salutation 'Namaste'.

Advait

Then interlace and bend the Ring fingers and the Little fingers of both the hands (see to it that the fingers are folded inwards, within the palms).

Extend out the Middle fingers and join the tips of both the Middle fingers and press slightly.

Now join the tips of the Index fingers to the tips of the Thumbs, forming interlocking circles (Refer the image).

This Mudra is to be held in front of your pubic bone.

While you are doing this Mudra, simultaneously keep contracting your Perineal floor muscle (Refer the image).

(Don't keep the muscle contracted but keep clenching and relaxing this muscle continuously)

Duration:

This Mudra should be performed till you feel tired by clenching and relaxing your Perineal muscle. Take rest then repeat a couple of times.

This Mudra should be performed twice a day, once in the morning and once in the evening for best results.

Benefits:

Mudras for Women

This Mudra is extremely beneficial in maintaining the health of our excretory system.

Its regular practice keeps the vital organs in our lower pelvic region in a healthy state.

This Mudra properly regulates the secretion of sexual hormones and plays a key role in maintaining fertility.

It is also used for treating hemorrhoids.

Mudra #16

Ushakaalmudra / Mudra of Morning

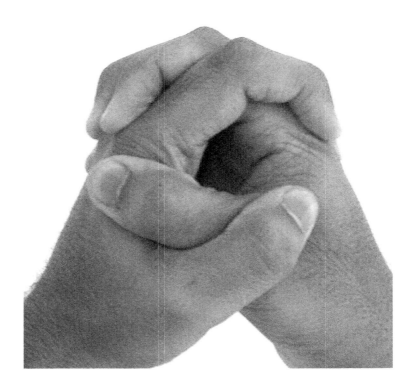

Method:

This Mudra can be performed while being seated,
in a standing position or lying in bed.

Mudras for Women

Concentrate on your breathing to relax and feel comfortable.

Clasp both your hands together as shown in the image.

Please note that the left index figure is on top of the right index finger.

Now, bring the tips of the Index finger and Thumb of the respective hands closer, but do not let them touch, simply form an open circle.

Duration:

This mudra should be performed for 5-10 minutes.

Benefits:

This is an extremely useful Mudra if you want to make a habit for waking up early for exercise and workout.

This mudra awakens the body and mind in morning hours.

**NOTE

Its name literally means 'The Mudra of the Morning'; it's a Mudra which induces alertness and vitality. It is advised that this Mudra should

Advait

be practiced daily when you wake up. Make a habit of performing this as a ritual when you awaken from your sleep.

***Important

Best results are achieved when this Mudra is performed facing the rising sun.

When you will perform this Mudra in the morning for the first time, you will feel an instant alertness induced as if you have just had a cup of espresso, this Mudra is that effective.

Mudra #17

Shanmukhamudra / Mudra of Six Faces

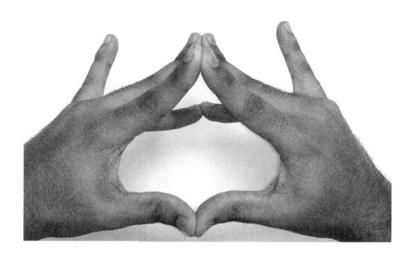

Method:

This Mudra is to be performed in a seated position.

Be seated comfortably in an upright posture and concentrate on your breathing to relax.

Hold your palms in front of your chest facing each other.

Now extend all the fingers on both the hands outwards.

Advait

Then, touch tips of all fingers of one hand to the tips of the respective fingers of the other hand, except the ring fingers.

Keep both the Ring fingers extended outwards.

(Refer the image)

Once the Mudra is formed lower the Mudra hold it in front of your abdomen.

Duration:

This Mudra should be performed for at least 5 minutes and can be performed for 40 minutes at a stretch.

This Mudra should be performed twice a day, once in the morning and once in the evening for best results.

Benefits:

This Mudra is extremely effective in maintaining the health of your hair.

Its regular practice stimulates and awakens our bodies self-healing potential.

It is also useful in strengthening ones bones.

Its regular practice also contributes towards enhancing our immune system.

Mudra #18

Pratham Yonimudra / Mudra of Vulva I

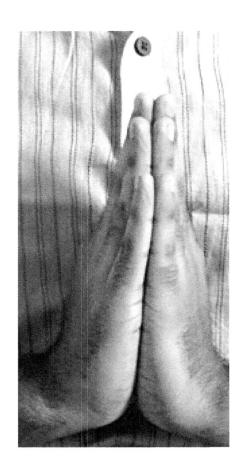

Mudras for Women

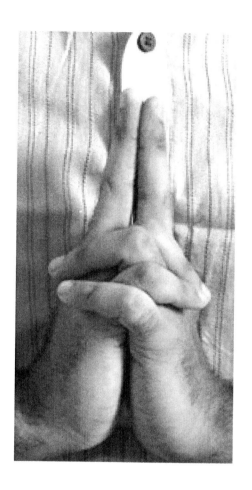

Advait

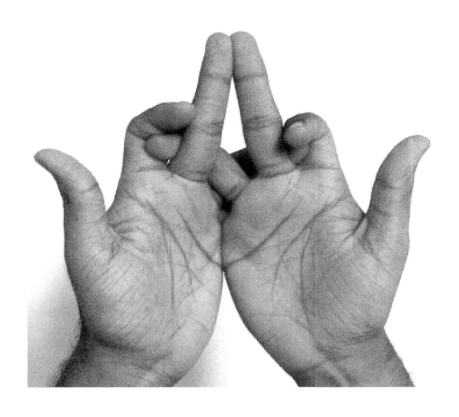

Mudras for Women

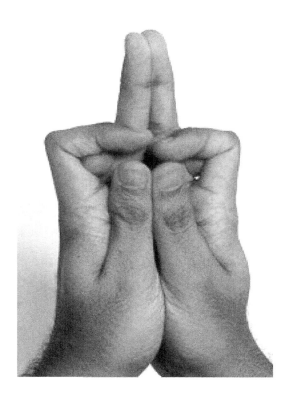

Method:

This Mudra has to be performed in a seated position.

Be seated comfortably in an upright posture and concentrate on your breathing to relax.

Join both the palms together like in the Indian salutation 'Namaste'.

Then interlace and bend the Ring fingers and the Little fingers of both the hands.

Advait

Now open the palms as if you are opening a pamphlet.

After you perform this, the tips of your Ring fingers will be forced into the openings between your Middle and Index fingers.

Now, press this tips of the Ring fingers down by the padding of your bent index fingers.

Close the palms together, and keep the Thumbs upright and parallel to each other.

This Mudra is to be held in front of the chest or pelvis.

For more clarification see the images provided.

Duration:

This Mudra should be performed for at least 5 minutes and can be performed for 20 minutes at a stretch.

This Mudra should be performed twice a day, once in the morning and once in the evening for best results.

Benefits:

This Mudra helps in improving the health of the sexual organs.

Mudras for Women

After performing this Mudra regularly you will observe an increase in natural lubrication during the act of sex.

Also this Mudra has been observed to enhance emotional sensitivity.

This Mudra is known to strengthen your connection with the divine feminine.

Advait

Mudra #19

Dwitiiya Yonimudra / Mudra of Vulva II

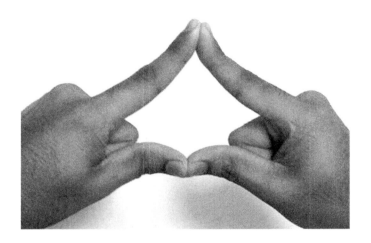

Method:

This Mudra has to be performed in a seated position.

Be seated comfortably in an upright posture and concentrate on your breathing to relax.

Outstretch the Index finger and the Thumb of both the hands.

Mudras for Women

Now, join the tip of the right Index finger to the tip of the left Index finger and the tip of the right Thumb to the tip of the Left Thumb. (You will form a triangular shape as shown in the image.)

The remaining three fingers of both the palms should be folded into the palm.

This Mudra has to be held in front of your pelvic region.

keep the index fingers pointing downwards. (Feminine Variation)

Duration:

This Mudra should be performed for 10 minutes. (5 minutes for the 1st variation and 5 minutes for the 2nd variation)

Benefits:

This Mudra revitalizes the pelvic and reproductive organs.

This Mudra is the one which connect your sexual energy to your spiritual energy.

This Mudra is also known as the connector between your creative energy and the divine.

Advait

Mudra #20

Tritiiya Yonimudra / Mudra of Vulva III

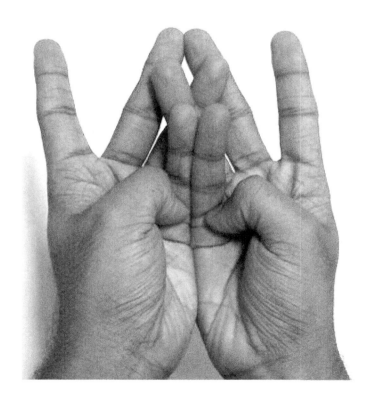

Method:

Mudras for Women

This Mudra has to be performed in a seated position.

Be seated comfortably in an upright posture and concentrate on your breathing to relax.

Keep your palms touching each other adjacently and facing you.

Cross the Ring finger of the right hand over the Ring finger of the left hand.

Join the tips of both the Middle fingers to each other.

Both the Little fingers should be pressed against each other adjacently.

Both the Index fingers should be stretched out pointing upwards.

This Mudra should be held in front of your chest.

Duration:

This Mudra should be performed for at least 5 minutes and can be performed for 25 minutes at a stretch.

This Mudra should be performed twice a day, once in the morning and once in the evening for best results.

Advait

Benefits:

This Mudra is extremely helpful in maintaining the health of your sexual and reproductive glands.

 This Mudra also enhances the luster of skin and lips.

This Mudra strengthens the kidneys and bladder.

Mudra #21

Sumukhmudra / Mudra of the Divine Face

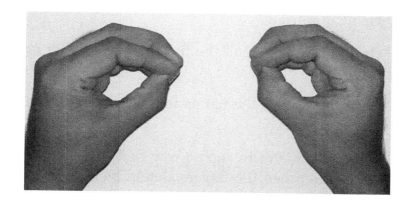

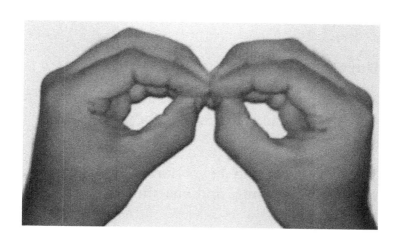

Advait

Method:

This Mudra has to be performed in a seated position.

Be seated comfortably in an upright posture and concentrate on your breathing to relax.

Keep your hands resting on your knees, palms facing upward.

On each hand join all the five fingers together at their tips.

Then bring both the hands together as shown in the image above.

Hold this mudra in such a way that the point of contact between the fingers should be directly in front of your sternum. (point at the end of your rib cage and start of your stomach).

Duration:

This Mudra should be performed for at least 5 minutes and can be performed for 30 minutes at a stretch.

This Mudra should be performed twice a day, once in the morning and once in the evening for best results.

Benefits:

This Mudra is used to attain a perfect balance between all the 5 elements that make up the human body.

This Mura when performed regularly harmonizes the body and brings a balance between different organs in the body.

This Mudra is useful in strengthening the tendons and ligaments in our limbs.

It is also known to stimulate our bodies self-healing capacity.

Mudra #22

SvadhishtaanaChakramudra / Mudra of Pelvic Centre Chakra

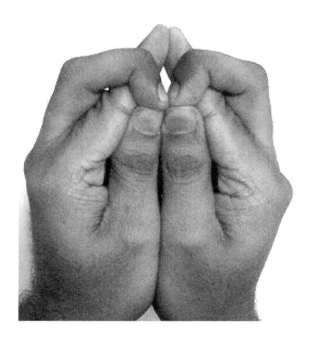

Method:

This Mudra can be performed while being seated, in a standing position or lying in bed.

Mudras for Women

Concentrate on your breathing to relax and feel comfortable.

Join both the palms together like in the Indian salutation 'Namaste'.

Then interlace and bend the Ring fingers and the Little fingers of both the hands within the palms.

Cross the Middle fingers over the Index fingers.

Touch the tip of the Middle fingers to the tip of the Thumbs and press slightly.

Press the heels of both the palms together.

Hold this Mudra in front of your chest.

Duration:

This Mudra should be performed for at least 5 minutes and can be performed for 30 minutes at a stretch.

This Mudra should be performed twice a day, once in the morning and once in the evening for best results.

Benefits:

This Mudra is known to open up our creative and spiritual capabilities.

Advait

Its regular practice purifies the blood.

It is also known to enhance ones fertility and sexual health.

Mudra #23

Tritiiya Varahamudra / Mudra of Hog
III

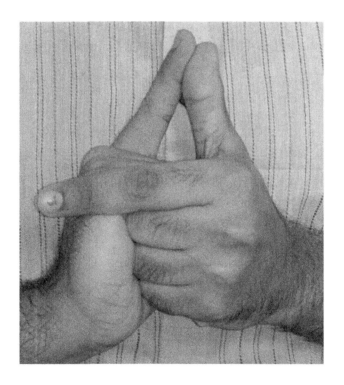

Method:

This Mudra is to be performed in a seated position.

Advait

Be seated comfortably in an upright posture and concentrate on your breathing to relax.

Hold your left hand in front of your chest, palm facing you.

Curl the Middle, Ring and Little finger of the left hand inwards.

The Index finger should be pointing towards right and the Thumb should be extended upwards.

Now, clasp the curled fingers of the left hand with the fingers of the right hand.

Then, touch the tip of the Thumb of your left hand with the tip of the Index finger of your right hand.

Touch the tip of your right Thumb to the base of the left Thumb.

The Left Index finger should be resting outside the right Little finger.

Duration:

This Mudra should be performed for at least 5 minutes and can be performed for 40 minutes at a stretch.

This Mudra should be performed twice a day, once in the morning and once in the evening for best results.

Mudras for Women

Benefits:

This is a very effective self-healing Mudra for various emotional problems.

It also induces a feeling of confidence and courage in the practitioner.

Mudra #24

Shankhamudra / Conch Mudra

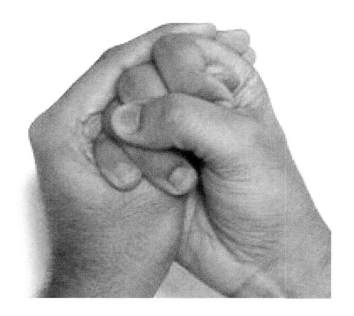

Method:

Make a fist with your right hand.

Insert the thumb of your left hand into that fist.

Flatten the rest of the four fingers of the left hand on the fist.

Now touch the tip of the index finger of the left hand, with the tip of the thumb of the right hand.

This will form a *Shankha*/Conch like structure.

Refer the above image for more clarity.

After 2.5 minutes exchange the Hands.

(Perform this Mudra by holding the hands in front of your chest)

Duration:

For 5 minutes at a time, for at least 3 times a day.

Benefits:

This Mudra is for curing problems with your voice.

This Mudra is effective in Tracheal, Thyroid and Tonsils disorders.

This Mudra also has an effect on the stomach; it aids in digestion, and helps in various intestinal disorders.

Advait

Mudra #25

Mahatrikamudra / Mudra of The Great Trinity

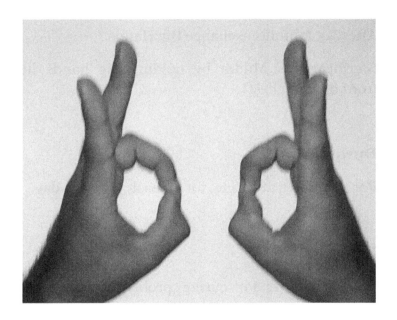

Mudras for Women

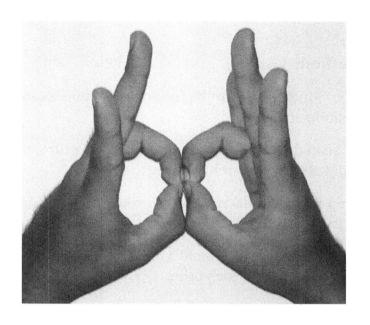

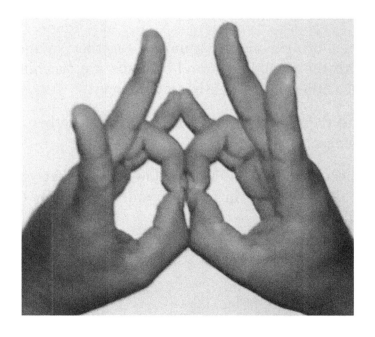

Advait

Method:

This Mudra has to be performed in a seated position.

Be seated comfortably in an upright posture and concentrate on your breathing to relax.

Keep your hands resting on your knees, palms facing upward.

After a few breaths, hold your palms in front of your neck, facing each other.

Join the tip of the ring finger and Thumb on each hand, To form a union of these two fingers on each hand. (refer image 1)

Then bring both these unions together so that both the ring fingers and Thumbs are touching each other. Press slightly. (refer image 2)

And then join both your little fingers together at the tips.

Once you form the Mudra, lower it so that you hold this Mudra in front of your lower belly or pubic bone.

Duration:

This Mudra should be performed for at least 5 minutes and can be performed for 15 minutes at a stretch.

This Mudra should be performed twice a day, once in the morning and once in the evening for best results.

Benefits:

This Mudra is extremely effective in regulating the menstrual cycle in women.

It also provides instant relief from menstrual cramps.

It is also useful in reliving pelvic congestion.

Advait

Mudras for Women

My Other Books on Mudras

Mudras for Awakening Chakras: 19 Simple Hand Gestures for Awakening & Balancing Your Chakras

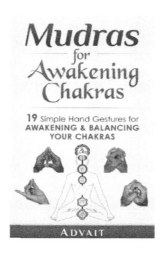

http://www.amazon.com/dp/B00P82COAY

[#1 Bestseller in 'Yoga']

[#1 Bestseller in 'Chakras']

Mudras for Weight Loss: 21 Simple Hand
Gestures for Effortless Weight Loss

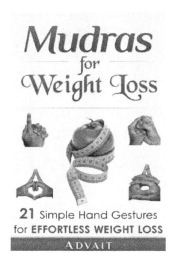

http://www.amazon.com/dp/B00P3ZPSEK

Mudras for Women

Mudras for Spiritual Healing: 21 Simple Hand Gestures for Ultimate Spiritual Healing & Awakening

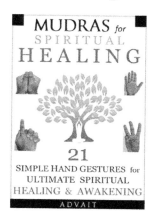

http://www.amazon.com/dp/B00PFYZLQO

Advait

Mudras for Sex: 25 Simple Hand Gestures for
Extreme Erotic Pleasure & Sexual Vitality

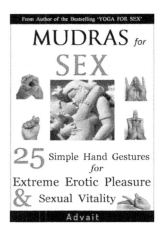

http://www.amazon.com/dp/B00OJR1DRY

Mudras for Women

Mudras: 25 Ultimate techniques for Self Healing

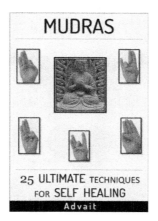

http://www.amazon.com/dp/B00MMPB5CI

Mudras for a Strong Heart: 21 Simple Hand
Gestures for Preventing, Curing & Reversing
Heart Disease

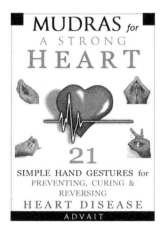

http://www.amazon.com/dp/B00PFRLGTM

Mudras for Women

Mudras for Anxiety: 25 Simple Hand Gestures for
Curing Your Anxiety

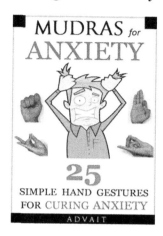

http://www.amazon.com/dp/B00PF011IU

Advait

Mudras for Memory Improvement: 25 Simple Hand Gestures for Ultimate Memory Improvement

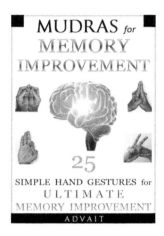

Mudras for Women

Mudras for Stress Management: 21 Simple Hand
Gestures for a Stress Free Life

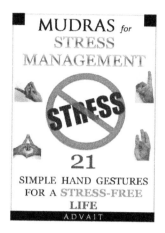

http://amazon.com/dp/B00PFTJ6OC

Advait

Mudras for Curing Cancer: 21 Simple Hand
Gestures for Preventing & Curing Cancer

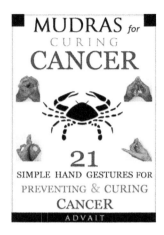

http://www.amazon.com/dp/B00PFO199M

Mudras for Women

Books by Advait on Yoga

Easy Yoga: Your Ultimate Beginners Guide to Understanding Yoga and Leading a Disease-Free Life through Routine Yoga Practice

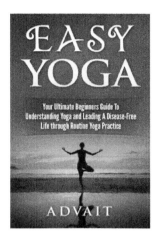

http://www.amazon.com/dp/B010I97366

Monday Yoga: Pranayam and Sukshma-Asana's for starting Your Routine Yoga Practice and Inducing Vigor into Your Life on the first day of the Week

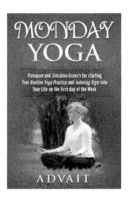

http://www.amazon.com/dp/B011SI6MK4

(This book is available for FREE)

Mudras for Women

Tuesday Yoga: 12 Yoga Asanas to be performed on
Tuesday as a Part of Your Daily Yoga Routine

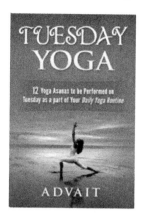

http://www.amazon.com/dp/B013GGA1AS

Advait

Wednesday Yoga: 12 Yoga Asanas to be performed on Wednesday as a Part of Your Daily Yoga Routine

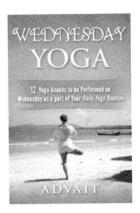

http://www.amazon.com/dp/B014RTDQ5U

Mudras for Women

Thursday Yoga: 12 Yoga Asanas to be performed on Thursday as a Part of Your Daily Yoga Routine

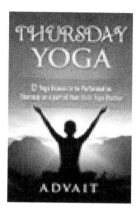

http://www.amazon.com/dp/B015JMSEPQ

Advait

Friday Yoga: 12 Yoga Asanas to be performed on
Friday as a Part of Your Daily Yoga Routine

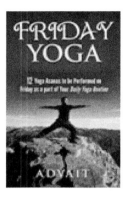

http://www.amazon.com/dp/B015UK17KG

Mudras for Women

Saturday Yoga: 12 Yoga Asanas to be Performed on Saturday as a Part of Your Daily Yoga Routine

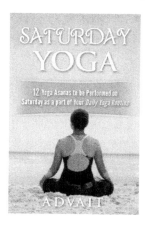

http://www.amazon.com/dp/B0165WFUJW

Advait

Sunday Yoga: Suryanamaskar (Sun Salutation) &
5 Yoga Asanas for a Blissful Culmination of Your
Daily Yoga Routine

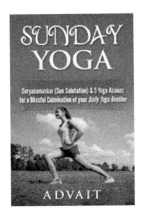

http://www.amazon.com/dp/B016Q8GF8K

Mudras for Women

Notes

Notes

Printed in Great Britain
by Amazon

37774223R00067